LOSE WEIGHT ONCE AND FOR ALL:

SOLUTIONS FOR PERMANENT WEIGHT LOSS

NICHOLAS M. EVANS

Table of Contents

INTRODUCTION

If you somehow happened to do an inquiry on long-lasting weight reduction, you'll find a variety of articles that will let you know it's reasonably unthinkable. They'll let you know extremely durable weight reduction is a fantasy, and the main way it's conceivable is with intrusive strategies like weight reduction medical procedures. While the facts confirm that roughly 95% of the time we restore our weight, it's generally a result of the techniques we are utilizing to lose that weight.

Food not just gives us the energy to get past our days, yet in addition a solace to a significant number of us. Be that as it may, it tends to be difficult to oppose food and quit eating when we're fully in the light of multiple factors

There's a great deal of joy that accompanies enjoying your number one tidbit or getting comfortable for a good, warm dinner. However, halting when you're full is an issue that a significant number of us face.

Fulfilling hunger is consistently something worth being thankful for, however a large number of us battle to check when we've had enough, driving us to indulge and try and put on weight in some cases.

If your technique for shedding pounds is through outrageous slimming down, you frequently lose a great deal of weight in a brief timeframe. Naturally, we as people are fretful. Regardless of whether you know it's not serving you; the convenient solution claim is difficult to avoid. It's exceptionally persuading when you see those individuals out there that seem, by all accounts, to find success with business diet programs and have these astonishing groundbreakings when photographs. The issue with this is that the speedier you lose, the faster you likewise recover the weight. That is the part you don't find in the titles or tributes. Thus, don't be tricked into thinking every other person has everything sorted out and you are fizzling.

CHAPTER ONE (1)

WHY YOUR BODY IS GENERALLY RAVENOUS

If horrible weight has left you hungrier than any time in recent memory, there is a purpose for it. As per a review distributed in the American Journal of Physiology, Endocrinology, and Metabolism, keeping a sound load after significant weight reduction can be hard. The examination concentrated on hunger in patients who partook in a complete two-year get-healthy plan and tracked down signs with regards to why keeping up with weight reduction long haul is so troublesome. Following two years, all the review members had shed pounds; be that as it may, the majority of them felt hungrier than when they had begun. The key seems, by all accounts, to be yet to be determined among craving and satiety chemicals in individuals who have lost very some weight. According to scientists, when we get in shape, the stomach discharges more prominent measures of a chemical called ghrelin, which causes us to feel hungry. Each individual has this chemical and if you are overweight and, get more fit, the chemical level increments. The degree of ghrelin doesn't change after some time. So fundamentally, individuals who have been overweight should manage expanded food cravings until the end of their lives because of this chemical.

According to the review, a corpulent individual has required more energy just to inhale, rest, digest food or walk. At the point when the body gets thinner, less energy is required for these fundamental capabilities, because the body is lighter then. Presently, somebody who has weighed 80 kilograms their entire life can eat more than 80 individual kilos in the wake of getting more fit. The distinction in how much food is around 400 calories and how much a decent breakfast or four bananas.

Fundamentally, individuals who have lost a critical measure of weight need less energy to keep up with their new and lighter bodies. But they feel hungrier because the body is attempting to get that load back.

CHAPTER TWO (2)

WHY DO YOU YIELD AND EAT "HORRENDOUS" (LOW QUALITY) FOOD?

At any point feel like you have an interminable desire for all the low-quality food — pungent, sweet, or both — that you can get your hands on?

You just really can't surrender it and continue eating, particularly during seasons of weighty pressure. What's more, there's unquestionably been a lot of pressure to keep us stirring things up around the town of chocolate the most recent a while.

"Particularly when we're anxious, low-quality food frequently calms us with minimal measure of quarrel and exertion. We search for sweet and greasy food sources to encourage us," says enlisted dietitian Beth Czerny, RD. "However, there are ways of dealing with your food desires, rather than them controlling you."

Is "unhealthy food" awful for you?

Low-quality food will be food that is undesirable for you, similarly to what "garbage" suggests. It runs the range from debilitated sweet (think: treats, treats, and cake) to weighty on soaked fats (think: broiled and handled food sources). Eating an excessive amount of low-quality food can have short-and long-haul ramifications for your body thanks to these fixings.

Soaked fats

Eating food sources wealthy in soaked fats can build your cholesterol levels and how much plaque is in your veins. "If you have veins that are solidifying and not moving blood really, you have a higher gamble for coronary illness, including cardiovascular failures and strokes," says Czerwony.

Sugars

A lot of sugar in your eating routine can prompt weight gain, a gamble factor for diabetes. A few creatures concentrate likewise propose that counterfeit sugars make our bodies oppose insulin. This may likewise improve the probability of creating prediabetes, diabetes, and coronary illness.

"Most Americans are strolling around with prediabetes, seriously jeopardizing them for creating Type 2 diabetes,"

Czerwony adds. "When you have diabetes, specialists treat you as though you've proactively had a cardiovascular failure because the pace of coronary illness is such a great deal higher. These medical problems influence every one of the organs, so making sense of them is significant."

What causes unhealthy food and sugar desires?

Czerwony records four reasons you might be needing desserts and other low-quality food.

1. Food rapture

Tragically, our bodies are permanently set up to pine for unhealthy food. At the point when you eat food varieties you appreciate, you animate the vibe great focuses in your cerebrum, setting off you to eat much more.

Particularly in patients with overabundance weight and stoutness, the mind's award handling framework for food resembles its systems connected with substance misuse. "Sugar makes us need to eat more sugar. Fat makes us need to eat more fat," notes Czerwony. "Our minds are pursuing that pleasurable condition of food rapture."

2. Absence of rest

Studies propose that lack of sleep is related to expanded hunger (particularly bite and sweet desires). What's more, you can pin it on your chemicals. The absence of rest causes chemical movements:

Ghrelin, the craving control chemical, increments, making you eat more.

Leptin, the hunger-smothering chemical, diminishes.

Cortisol, the pressuring chemical, may increment, invigorating your craving.

Research shows that lack of sleep causes an expansion in and large appetite, which can prompt desires for sugar, fat, or both.

3. Propensity

"Assuming it's typical for you to eat low-quality food, it tends to be difficult to break that cycle," makes sense of Czerwony. "You're utilized to not cooking, getting ready, or arranging. You eat anything available because that you've generally finished."

4. Stress

Stress, or profound, eating truly is a thing — and it's the consequence of both nature and support. Certain individuals find food occupies them from pessimistic considerations and sentiments. Others advanced as youngsters to utilize food to adapt.

Chemicals are additionally dependable. Like the absence of rest, continuous pressure makes the body increment levels of cortisol and different chemicals associated with hunger. Concentrates on showing this chemical tidal wave increments craving — alongside your longing for sweet and greasy food sources.

Seven methods for controlling low quality food desires

Czerwony says these techniques can assist you with dominating your food desires:

Practice care: Try to eat and drink without interruptions, Czerwony prompts: "Abstain from eating in the vehicle or while sitting in front of the TV or noting messages. Truly center around appreciating and tasting your food. You'll find that a couple of chomps can fulfill your desire — and save a ton of calories."

Attempt an air fryer: "One of the most incredible late creations is the convection air fryer. It permits you to eat things that have a broiled consistency, short the oil," makes sense of Czerwony. "It's a better method for reveling."

Embrace feast arranging: Czerwony says when you prepare, you engage yourself to use sound judgment. "Regardless of whether you pick a food that is not beneficial, it ought not to be an issue on the off chance that you plan for it by eating better for two or three days prior or later." Other ways of arranging to incorporate reserving solid snacks in your pack or work area and plan suppers early so your brain (and not your stomach) chooses the menu.

Give yourself non-food-related rewards: If treating yourself generally includes undesirable food sources, you could be attacking your wellbeing objectives. All things being equal, indulge yourself with another outfit, some spoiling, or another movement that makes you grin.

Hydrate: It's not difficult to mistake thirst signals for hunger desires. To remain hydrated the entire day, keep a water bottle reachable.

Get a decent night's rest: Keep those yearning chemicals under wraps with satisfactory rest.

Oversee pressure: "On the off chance that you develop a solid way of life, those desires frequently disappear because the body isn't answering pressure. Attempt contemplation, exercise, or perusing to settle yourself down in unpleasant minutes."

Czerwony additionally accentuates that it's OK to request help while you're feeling stuck. "Chat with your essential consideration doctor or an enrolled dietitian. That we're hanging around for: to teach and engage you to pursue better choices. We can assist you with picking better choices and changes instead of zeroing in on things you need to cut."

Solid choices to unhealthy food

At the point when you try to comprehend what flavors you do and could do without, finding better alternatives is simpler. Czerwony proposes a couple of suggestions to kick you off:

Same food, different adaptation

Take a stab at switching around the style of food rather than the actual food.

Attempt stove-prepared or air-broiled adaptations of your #1 seared food varieties.

Eat lower-sugar renditions of your number one treats and desserts — or stick to more modest segments.

Attempt pizza with 100 percent entire grain outside, either produced using scratch or at eateries that offer it. You can likewise make specialty outsides — produced using fixings like cauliflower. Also, don't hold back on the veggies!

Eat potatoes with the skin. The additional fiber in the potato skin eases back assimilation and keeps your glucose in balance.

Attempt this rather than that

Sort out an extraordinary change to move you along.

Have a chocolate-plunged pretzel or piece of the natural product rather than a whole chocolate bar.

In recipes, have a go at trading fruit purée for oil or diminishing sugar by something like one-fourth.

Next time you need a carbonated beverage, settle on shimmering water without sugar or fake sugars.

Trade out white potatoes for yams, which are lower on the glycemic record and higher in micronutrients.

Rather than pretzels and chips, appreciate air-popped popcorn, popcorn made with additional virgin olive oil, or unsalted blended nuts.

Take a stab at supplanting sweet treats with berries and dull chocolate (more than 70%). Add a touch of nut spread for protein and solid fat. Different choices incorporate berry natural teas, frozen berries, and custom-made nut balls improved with a few Medjool dates.

Opposing food desires are significant assuming you're attempting to get more fit or lessen circulatory strain or cholesterol. However, such an amazing concept is overall excessively prohibitive. "If you're moderately solid, at a sound weight, and your circulatory strain and glucose are spot on, go ahead and enjoy assuming you plan for it," Czerwony says.

"A significant number of my patients eat around their desire. At the point when they need something chocolatey, they eat a piece of natural product that doesn't raise a ruckus around town. Then they go for an ice pop with a similar outcome ... and it goes on," Czerwony says.

Simply eat what you're longing for, truly appreciate it, and be finished with it," she recommends. "Like that, you'll be fulfilled and won't have to return for more."

CHAPTER THREE (3)

THE MOST EFFECTIVE METHOD TO QUANTIFY GENUINE HUNGER

The main thing to overseeing weight is to eat less, yet not to feel ravenous or denied. Being ravenous all the time is capital punishment for any health improvement plan.

The longing to eat begins with a twinge, and in a flash, you're scrounging through the ice chest. Yet, the genuine inquiry is: Are you truly eager, or was that a twinge of propensity, fatigue, or another inclination? Understanding your dietary patterns and figuring out how to perceive genuine yearning is a fundamental weight reduction device.

The choice to eat is impacted by a large group of variables: sights, smells, and group environments, and that's just the beginning.

We eat to fulfill our cravings yet, in addition, to relieve feelings, celebrate triumphs, fulfill social assumptions - - and because it simply tastes great.

Researchers have been exploring the effects of cravings and long for many years. The body's frameworks are complicated. "Hunger chemicals" (ghrelin) in your blood and an unfilled stomach signal the cerebrum when you're ravenous. Nerves in the stomach convey messages to the cerebrum that you're full, however, these signs can require as long as 20 minutes to impart - - and at that point, you might have previously eaten excessively.

Rating Your Hunger

At the point when you plunk down to eat dinner, you need to be eager, yet entirely not greedy. (Allowing your blood to sugar get so low that you feel voracious frequently prompts pigging out.) And your objective is to stop when you're serenely full.

To start assessing your appetite, rate your craving and fulfillment level when each dinner. Here is a mathematical scale you could utilize:

1. Ravenously eager, salivating.

2. Hungry, paunch snarling.

3. Mildly eager; you might require a light nibble to hold you over, however, you could hold out somewhat longer.

4. Satisfied; don't have to eat any longer.

5. More than fulfilled; ate excessively.

6. Stuffed like a Thanksgiving turkey.

Also, at whatever point you're going to race to the kitchen or lunchroom or diversion to the closest drive-through, pose yourself these inquiries first:

When did I last eat? Assuming it was under 2-3 hours prior, you're presumably not feeling a genuine craving.

Might a little, nutritious nibble wealthy in fiber at some point hold you over until the following dinner?

Could you at any point drink a glass of water and stand by 20 minutes?

If you find that you don't effectively perceive the indications of appetite, plan your feasts and bites. Partition your eating plan into a few little dinners, dispersed each three to four hours. Rate your craving each time you plunk down to eat, and attempt to turn out to be more mindful of what a genuine appetite feels like.

More Mindful Eating

The majority of us wolf down our food without genuinely tasting it occasionally. Do you experience the ill effects of "eating amnesia" when the hand-to-mouth movement becomes programmed - - typically before the TV or while perusing a book? Negative behavior patterns are difficult to break, yet to control what you eat, you should turn out to be more aware of all that you put into your mouth.

It assists with dialing back and partaking in your dinners, as they do in France. Plunk down, switch off the TV, and establish a serene climate liberated from interruptions to enjoy your feasts.

Remember that the initial not many chomps are consistently awesome (your taste buds before long become less sharpened to the synthetic compounds in food that make it taste so great). Center around the nature of the food, not the amount. Be aware of every significant piece, and value the flavors, smells, and surfaces of the food.

Getting a charge out of relaxed dinners gives your stomach time to flag your mind that you are serenely full. Put your fork down between nibbles, taste water, and appreciate the discussion while you feast.

Manage Your Hunger

Here are a few additional tips to assist you with reaching out to genuine yearning:

Practice segment control. The adage "your appetite tends to take over" might be wise counsel. Specialist Barbara Rolls and her partners at Pennsylvania State University have observed that the more food you're served, the more you're probably going to eat. The hypothesis is that the ecological signs of part size abrogate the body's prompts of fulfillment.

Gobble food sources that are built up with water or air, give them more volume and make them seriously fulfilling. Expanding the mass in your feasts helps fill your stomach, signals satiety to your cerebrum, and permits you to feel full on fewer calories. Stock-based soups, stews, hot cereals, and cooked grains are genuine instances of food sources that take care of business.

Fiber can assist with fulfilling hunger and lessen craving. Pick high-fiber food varieties like organic products, vegetables, vegetables, popcorn, and entire grains. Beginning a feast with an enormous plate of mixed greens can assist you with eating fewer calories during dinner given the fiber and water content of greens and vegetables. Likewise, remember that new organic products have more fiber and water than dried ones.

Keep away from the smorgasbord line. At the point when there are loads of decisions, the vast majority eat more. Keep it basic, limit the number of courses, and top off on the high-fiber food sources first.

Remember lean protein for your feasts and snacks to assist them with enduring longer in your stomach. A modest bunch of nuts, some low-fat dairy, soy protein, or lean meat, fish, or chicken will hold you over for quite a long time.

Food wasn't at any point expected to be this precarious. Simply ask any crying infant. No doubt, she sounds hungry. She ought to eat.

Yet, for loads of reasons - from an over-burden of mind seizing sugar, salt, and fat in our food supply to our folks' benevolent propensity to "reward" us with treats when we were respectful - we've grown up to need food, when we're ravenous, however when we're exhausted, pushed, blissful, tired, dawdling or, hello, since we see a gelato and it looks pretty darn great.

"A great many people eat less nourishment for hunger than for these different reasons," says Dr. Michelle May, the pioneer behind Am I Hungry? careful eating projects and creator of "Eat What You Love, Love What You Eat." And while it's a commonplace piece of being human to eat only for delight from time to time, letting your craving as opposed to your yearning drive most of your food admission is an essential driver of weight gain and heftiness, she says.

The Beauty of Following Your Hunger Cues

"Figuring out how to recognize hunger prompts and eat in light of those signs, and not others, is a powerful method for getting in shape without counting calories," says enrolled dietitian Georgie Fear, creator of "Lean Habits for Lifelong Weight Loss." "Let your body crunch the numbers. It is more exact than any telephone application or distributed sustenance realities." Additionally, your craving will rise and fall with movement levels, so you don't need to stress over the amount to change your admission upwards when you take up tennis, or the amount to tone down if you break a leg and need to briefly surrender your climbing leisure activity. Your hunger will change as your requirements change, every day and week-to-week.

For example, in one Public Health Nutrition investigation of more than 1,600 moderately aged ladies, the people who ate in light of craving were bound to be at a solid weight contrasted with the individuals who didn't eat because of their yearning prompts. In the meantime, a 2014 survey of 26 examinations connected "natural eating" - that is, eating because of physiological yearning - with not simply a lower weight file, or BMI, (a marker of body creation), yet additionally bringing down pulse and cholesterol levels, better food decisions and worked on by and large wellbeing. "At the point when we eat for hunger, as opposed to for these different reasons, food can fill its actual need to support and fuel our bodies," May says.

Sadly, knowing precisely when you're eager is more earnestly than it sounds. "The counsel to eat when you're eager is beguilingly straightforward," May says. That is because we are in general so detached from our craving signals, familiar with eating because of reasons separated from hunger, that it tends to be difficult to determine what a valid, physiological appetite feels like.

Furthermore, people with a background marked by consuming fewer calories - particularly with very prohibitive or prevailing fashion slim down - can frequently have significantly more difficulty than most with regards to understanding their craving signals, she says. All things considered, hardship slims down, purges, and end counts calories frequently firmly control when and what you should eat. You eat when the eating routine says, not when you're eager. Since, can we just be real for a moment, on these eating regimens, you are ravenous constantly.

So Are You Hungry? Follow These Tips to Find Out

With regards to seeing whether you, as a matter of fact, really need to eat, the initial step is to stop and ask yourself, "Am I hungry?"

It sounds straightforward and perhaps a piece senseless, yet the basic inquiry is an entryway opener, May says. To arrive at a basic "yes" or "no" end, she suggests doing what she calls a body-mind-heart check, seeing what's happening in your body, both truly and inwardly. Is your stomach snarling? How are your energy levels? And your temperament? What were you doing when eating jumped into your head?

Run-of-the-mill side effects of genuine yearning and a need to eat incorporate food cravings, stomach snarling, and plunges in glucose, set apart by low energy, precariousness, migraines, and issues centering, as per Fear. "In any case, if you would turn down an apple, yet are still 'ravenous' enough to eat a piece of candy, you probably won't be feeling physiological yearning," she says. By taking into account all that is happening in your reality by then, you can begin to see every one of the elements that are impacting your outings to the kitchen, candy machine, or nibble cabinet.

May likens this sweep to checking your fuel measure when you pass a service station on the expressway. "You don't simply pull in," she says. You hope to perceive how much fuel you right now have in the tank, the number of miles that are between you and the following corner store, and perhaps consider the off chance that you want a restroom break before choosing whether to pull over.

This raises a valid statement: Even on the off chance that you choose you're not ravenous (think: fuel check on E), one choice is to feel free to eat, at any rate, May says. All things considered, perhaps your next valuable open door to eat won't introduce itself for an additional couple of hours, so you want to get in lunch while you can. Or on the other hand, you simply need to have a cut of birthday cake because, hello, it's your birthday! (Eating because of reasons like these once in a while is not a problem and an ordinary piece of adjusted eating. It's the point at which you surrender to non-hunger reasons constantly that you can cause problems.)

In any case, different choices include diverting your consideration, which proves to be useful when it's just a natural sign -, for example, strolling by a popcorn shop, hitting up a party with a smorgasbord table brimming with hors d'oeuvres or simply watching a truly enticing café business - that you choose is making you need to eat, she says. By possessing yourself briefly with exercises like conversing with a companion, watching an entertaining video cut, or simply browsing your email, you can take your brain off food sufficiently long to make your false craving blur. That's what the objective is, when you wrap up your interruption, your cerebrum doesn't jump back to harping on that messy popcorn.

In the meantime, assuming you conclude that your purposes behind needing to eat are feeling based, established in pressure, culpability, fatigue, nervousness, or dejection, keeping an eye on those feelings head-on can't forestall gorging - it can encourage better profound and emotional wellness.

"Commonly, when we assume we generally dislike food, our concerns are truly by the way we are meeting our feelings," May says. "By giving air to our sentiments and tending to them, we can meet our feelings better than we at any point could with food." (Don't stress on the off chance that you understand you're doing this; we all are close-to-home eaters partially.)

Thus, for example, when you understand you need to eat because you're exhausted, sort out why you're exhausted and afterward get a few social plans on the schedule, begin an undertaking at home, or search for a task that you see as really captivating, truly assists with taking care of the issue, as opposed to simply swathing it up with fat and sugar. As a figuring out how to designate or simply say "no" to projects that you lack opportunity and energy to take on, as opposed to stuffing your timetable - and your face - out of pressure.

Like May says, that basic inquiry, "Am I hungry?" is both misleading and straightforward (this truly takes some work!) and an entryway opener. Take it, however, and the progressions to your wellbeing, brain, and body will be in every way justified.

CHAPTER FOUR (4)

INVESTIGATING - WEIGHT LOSS TROUBLE AND HOW TO SETTLE THEM

Assuming that you've encountered boundaries to weight reduction, you're in good company. Everybody encounters difficulties that are well defined for their singular weight reduction venture. Your life conditions, stress, funds, time, hereditary qualities, and self-perception can all become obstructions to sound weight reduction, however, that doesn't mean you can't pursue beating them.

A great many people can hope to experience road obstructions while attempting to arrive at their weight reduction objectives. The people who are effective at getting thinner and keeping it off are the ones who figure out how to get through their weight reduction obstructions as they emerge.

Distinguishing Weight Loss Barriers

The initial step is to search inside. Realize that a significant number of the difficulties you're confronting have been looked at previously. Eating invigoratingly and adhering to an activity program isn't simply all of the time. A great many people experience highs and lows en route. When you perceive your obstructions, you can foster the ability to transcend them.

Some weight reduction hindrances are seen as boundaries, implying that the obstruction depends on your viewpoints or sentiments. Seen boundaries can be similarly just about as huge and genuine as substantial hindrances, which can incorporate ailments and actual limits. Whether your difficulties are seen or concrete, most can be grouped into three primary classifications: physical, ecological, and profound.

Actual Barriers to Weight Loss

Normal actual obstructions to weight reduction incorporate weariness, distress, and hidden clinical issues. Issues, for example, parchedness and absence of rest may likewise assume a part in your capacity to get in shape. While these obstructions can be huge, there are ways of getting around them regardless get in shape.

Speak With Your Physician

Converse with your PCP about your battles to get thinner. Maybe there is a clinical issue adding to your disappointment.

For instance, certain drugs (counting steroids, contraception pills, and a few antidepressants) can cause weight gain. If you have as of late stopped smoking, you might encounter weight gain.

Hormonal changes (like those accomplished during menopause) may make weight reduction more troublesome and add to weight gain. Ailments including PCOS and certain thyroid problems are related to weight gain.

9 Reasons You May Be Gaining Weight

Grow Your Healthcare Team

Ask you're essential consideration doctor for references to an enrolled dietitian, actual advisor, therapist, or potentially corpulence medication subject matter expert. These experts can fit your treatment program to help your objectives.

With a doctor's reference, there is normally a superior opportunity that administrations will be covered by protection. Look at your approach to find what your arrangement will cover. Talk with the expert's office to inquire as to whether required.

Work on Your Sleep

Analysts have found that not getting sufficient rest can disturb your digestion. Your hormonal equilibrium can move when you don't get the rest you want, and you might encounter expanded hunger and appetite.1 as a matter of fact, proof shows that individuals who get less complete long periods of rest (under seven hours) are bound to be overweight or have obesity.2

Fortunately rolling out a couple of improvements to your rest routine might assist you with arriving at your weight reduction objectives. Specialists prescribe that you nod off simultaneously every evening, rest in a cool, dull room, and eliminate electronic gadgets, (for example, tablets and mobile phones) to empower a loosening up the climate.

Get Hydrated

Basic changes to your everyday schedule can make weight reduction more straightforward. Remaining hydrated is one straightforward change that has various medical advantages. Studies have shown that drinking more water is related to better weight reduction results.3

Confounding the impressions of appetite and thirst is generally to be expected. Keep filled water bottles in your cooler to get in and out. Add berries or different fixings (like basil or cucumber) on the off chance that you incline toward seasoned drinks. Assuming you wind up brushing in the kitchen over the day, think about drinking a few ounces of water before eating to check whether it fulfills your hankering.

Make Flavored Water Recipes with Fewer Calories

Get Your Work done

Research different activity plans and sound cooking tips. Propensities that lead to weight reduction are more reasonable when they're entertaining. For instance, non-weight-bearing exercises, like water heart stimulating exercise, might be more agreeable on the off chance that you have stoutness, torment, or joint issues.

Make changes to your everyday dinner plan by pursuing an enlightening cooking class where you can learn better approaches to get ready vegetables or lean meats and partake in your time in the kitchen.

Ecological Barriers to Weight Loss

At the point when your environmental elements don't uphold a sound eating regimen and exercise plan, it can feel like you're wasting time and energy. Ecological obstructions, including restricted admittance to good food or exercise offices, unfortunate social help, or an absence of time because of social, family, and expert tensions can cause weight reduction to appear to be incomprehensible.

Converse with the People Around You

Get support from loved ones by imparting your necessities. Be explicit about the manners in which they can assist with making your arrangement a triumph. Perhaps your accomplice will take on additional errands, or your children could assist more around the house.

Your boss may uphold your solid way of life by offering health assets or adaptability in your plan for getting work done. A better worker is a more useful representative. Fortunately, an ever-increasing number of businesses have started perceiving the advantages of health programs.

Get Creative with Exercise

If going to the exercise center is impossible for you, a lot of at-home exercise choices are accessible. You can find free exercises on the web (actually take a look at YouTube or Instagram). There are additionally a lot of cell phone and tablet applications that give practice programming. You'll track down various sorts of classes as well as tips, discussions, and different assets.

You can likewise exploit the assets just beyond your doorstep to get in shape. Strolling is a magnificent method for working out. Stroll on neighborhood ways, climb the steps in your office or high rise, or plan a family climb throughout the end of the week. Many shopping centers offer exceptional hours for walkers who need to practice before the groups dominate.

Profound Barriers to Weight Loss

It sounds irrational to say that you need to shed pounds, yet your sentiments about weight reduction keep you down. In any case, close-to-home boundaries to weight reduction are factual and frequently critical. These boundaries might incorporate incredulity about your capacity to arrive at your objectives, a negative relationship with actual work, high feelings of anxiety, or an absence of inspiration.

Enroll with the Help of a Qualified Professional

Numerous conduct wellbeing subject matter experts (counting social specialists, advisors, and clinicians) center around the feelings connected with body weight. If you have proactively researched conceivable clinical explanations behind your weight concerns, think about addressing a specialist regarding close-to-home worries.

Figure out how to Motivate Yourself

Inspiration is an expertise that you can master. Strategies like positive self-talk and journaling are demonstrated to help your inspiration levels and power you forward in the correct heading.

Self-observing has likewise been displayed as a successful device for weight loss.4 Self-checking might incorporate keeping a food journal, standard weigh-ins, or following your active work with a paper log or an application. Self-checking assists you with noticing your everyday ways of behaving to expand attention to make changes depending on the situation.

Step-by-step instructions to Motivate Yourself for Weight Loss

Use Stress-Reduction Techniques

Stress — connected with your bustling timetable, family issues, an absence of weight reduction results, or a continuous ailment — can rapidly prompt profound eating and weight gain. Constant pressure is related to obesity.5

Then again, stress decrease procedures (like profound breathing or directed representation) have been displayed to further develop weight reduction outcomes.6 Learn pressure decrease systems like breathing strategies, reflection, or journaling. Plan these exercises into your day to save yourself the right attitude for progress.

Profound Barriers to Weight Loss

Keep in mind, that accomplishing and keeping a solid weight is a long-distance race, not a run. Similarly, that one day of good dieting will not fix a month of fewer sound decisions, the opposite is likewise evident.

Make the most of chances in your everyday life to go with nutritious decisions. Offsetting your way of life with customary actual work and stress the board methods can go quite far in feeling your best at any weight.

ANSWERS FOR WEIGHT LOSS CHALLENGES

Assisting individuals with carrying on with better lives is my thing. As I frequently get the chance to visit with a large number of you and catch wind of the difficulties you face in attempting to get thinner, I chose to gather together the hindrances to weight reduction I find out about most frequently, and share my best arrangements with you. How about we start with this: you are not taking on the weight reduction conflict alone. Bunches of individuals share comparative battles, and I am hanging around for you! The following are 11 answers to the most well-known weight reduction challenges.

1. Nothing is working.

You've attempted everything. You further developed your dietary patterns and you work out routinely. The main thing that will not coordinate is your scale. You are caught in a weight reduction level and you've not been persuaded the scale will at any point dive in the future. If you are burnt out on seeing similar three numbers on the scale, attempt this:

Arrangement: If what you are doing isn't working, change what you are doing. OK, I realize that is Captain Obvious, yet here and there an update is useful. Change your exercise. Change the sort, power, and span. Assuming all you are hitting the treadmill, add some strength preparing. Add greater development to your day on top of ordinary activity. Stand more. Move more. Walk more advances. Recall that you can't simply practice your direction to your ideal weight, you need to wed it with good dieting. Get away from inexpensive food, handled food, and eat clean. Also, watch those bits. Segment control is so significant.

2. I could do without working out.

I generally laugh a smidgen when I hear this since there are such countless types of activity ... would you say you are truly saying you like NONE of them? Truly? The uplifting news is you don't need to go through your time on earth working out; you simply have to commit around four percent of your 24-hour day to the reason.

Arrangement: There must be something you like. Dance? Swimming? Strolling? Nia? The treadmill? A gathering wellness classes? Cycling? Or on the other hand what might be said about attempting a virtual exercise? Commit a month to attempt all types of activity as an examination until you land on one you love. Reward tip: Sometimes a music playlist you love can be exactly what you want to cherish your exercise.

3. I lack the opportunity.

Indeed, who does? In the first place, let me give you a major embrace. Presently for genuine affection: "I lack the opportunity" is only a reason and a snag. By utilizing this famous reason, you can continuously legitimize not working out. What's more, it's an extreme one to defeat except if you let go of it completely because when do you simply awaken and have the entire day free? To start with, focus on at no point ever expressing this in the future, and afterward do this ...

Arrangement: Two words: Schedule it. That's right. Do you know how you plan your arrangement with the dental specialist? Or then again, an arrangement to finish your hair? Plan your activity very much like that — make it an arrangement. Simply ensure you do it more frequently than once at regular intervals. Truly, however, booking it is the best way to get it going. You are an incredible CEO, so immediate your day to get practice going. Furthermore, stop and think for a minute, when you get the energy of activity moving and into an ordinary mood, it will be hard for you NOT to work out.

4. I have a physical issue that keeps me from doing particular sorts of activity.

Loads of individuals have knee issues and back issues and different issues that can keep them from doing specific activities, similar to the bouncing found with plyometric practices or the beating from running. Be that as it may, there are countless ways of stilling get development into your day.

Arrangement: First, check with your primary care physician for endorsed works out. Your physical issue type will figure out what you should or shouldn't do, however strolling is in many cases an activity that the vast majority can in any case do. Many individuals with knee issues can profit from an exercise bike and I love doing yoga and board activities to assist with my back issues. Simply recall there's dependably a workaround so doesn't abandon practice since you have a physical issue.

5. I can't bear the cost of exercise center participation at present.

Not all exercise centers are economical and I get that, however, this is the age of everything computerized. You simply need to know where to look.

Arrangement: If the exercise center close to you seems like the expense of a nation club participation, recall that you can get reasonable exercises from me! That's right, look at our Exercise Library here. Bunches of moves you can manage without going out. Also, look at getting Healthy U TV, my freshest exercise site. You can approach every one of my exercises for a month-to-month charge and stream them on any gadget or your TV.

a beautiful lady doing practices on her yoga mat at home

6. I gorge on parties.

At the point when individuals let me know they gorge at parties as a result of the enticing procession of food directly in front of them, I ask them what they ate before the party. Most frequently, individuals go on a small-scale starvation diet earlier paving the way to the party thinking they are saving calories for some other time. That is presumably the most exceedingly terrible thing you can do because you are showing up for a party with a covetous stomach. Do this all things being equal ...

Arrangement: Eat a protein nibble before the party. Showing up at a party hungry scramble your great judgment. If you have a small bunch of nuts before a party, your hunger will be satisfied to where you can go with savvy decisions about testing your top choices and not eating up two platefuls of party food sources.

7. I feel constrained to eat with my loved ones.

Whether it's your mother, your grandma, or the most loved pastry specialist in your family, there's generally somebody who is attempting to show their affection by taking care of you. It's sweet, yet it very well may be hard to explore obligingly on the off chance that you are attempting to control the amount you eat.

Arrangement: If you are gifted with sweet treats, share the adoration with other relatives and companions. If you are at an evening gathering and you don't need seconds, simply be thoughtful and direct. Attempt a "Gracious, it was so great and I'm so full, I just could never have another nibble." Try and recall the vast majority mean well and are simply attempting to fulfill you with food. They aren't attempting to disrupt your weight. On the off chance that you truly do think somebody is attempting to obstruct the entirety of your persistent effort, read our article about food pushers.

8. I simply don't have inspiration.

You simply don't awaken with a flash or a fire to destroy the exercise center. You see others truly into it however it's simply not you. You even wish you were loaded with inspiration to burn the calories, however, nothing truly does it for you. What do you do?

Arrangement: If you don't have the inspiration, yet you need to track down the inspiration, that is a decent beginning. Distinguish your greatest WHY. What's the one explanation you need to carry on with a solid life? Is it for personal satisfaction? To live to the extent that this would be possible? To be more fearless? To like garments once more? To have more energy? Get clear on your main motivation to get sound and afterward mortar it on a piece of paper where you can peruse it every day. My next best inspiration tip is this: Just phony it tills you make it. Now and again, it's the stalling began that keeps us out. When you start, it's a lot more straightforward to move that magic along!

9. I eat extraordinary the entire day and afterward ruin my extraordinary choices around evening time with nibbling.

Evening time accompanies a couple of difficulties for the vast majority. Once in a while, it's the time when you ease the pressure. In some cases, it's the point at which the TV comes on and your butt gets on the love seat. Can we just be real, it's amusing to nibble, and assuming we have supper at 6, we can get eager again at 9 PM. So how would we avoid the storage room?

Arrangement: Eat a sound bite that tops you off. Try not to think you need to quit eating for four hours before you hit the sack. Simply pick a nibble shrewdly. One of my top picks is smooth Greek yogurt for certain frozen berries and a few nuts like pecans or almonds. It's tasty and can thoroughly control my hunger from nibbling or returning to the storage space on various occasions. Another of my go-to snacks is sound air-popped popcorn (not the microwave-in-a-pack stuff). Popcorn is brimming with fiber; it fills the need to crunch alongside your number one show and it won't impair you in calories.

10. I very much like sugar excessively.

Ahhhh, the sweet tooth. I have one as well. It can truly undermine your endeavors assuming you experience difficulty controlling your bits. My most memorable recommendation is to quit thinking you need to remove all sugar to hit your objective weight. You don't need to go virus on sugar. Simply do this all things considered ...

Arrangement: obviously, you need to watch segments to shed pounds, however, you don't need to surrender sugar or overlook your sweet tooth. Make better sweets all things considered. I have heaps of better treats on my site Get Healthy U for nothing. Figure out how to make each of your top choices somewhat better.

11. Practicing good eating habits is costly.

Indeed, it tends to be nevertheless it doesn't need to be. There are heaps of workarounds!

Arrangement: Eat food varieties that are in season. At the point when certain foods grown from the ground are in season, they are more affordable. Assuming some new product is still too expensive, (similar to berries) pick frozen produce. It's more affordable yet sound. Heaps of food sources you can purchase at the store are more affordable assuming you make them yourself like kale chips or energy bars.

What's your greatest test for weight reduction? We should make a big difference in the discussion! Your answer is standing by!

CHAPTER FIVE (5)

MAKING YOUR UNIQUE EATING PLAN

Arranging can truly assist you with having quality dinners and snacks regardless of how occupied things get.

Arranging can assist you with having quality feasts and snacks regardless of how occupied things get. Having a dinner plan can save time, and cash and diminish food squander. Simply make sure to adhere to your shopping list.

The following are six moves toward making a feast arrangement:

1. allow yourself to design

Put away the opportunity every week to make a feast arrangement. Contemplate:

The number of dinners you need to plan for the week

At the point when you want to make speedy feasts or set them up ahead of time

2. Check what you have

Check what fixings you as of now have in your pantry, refrigerator, or cooler. Look at the 'utilization by' dates of food sources to see what you want to go through first, begin by arranging your dinners around this. Peruse additional shopping tips here

How you store food hugely affects how long it endures. Follow these tips:

Look at the name for counsel on the best way to store food.

Put new things to the back, and more established things to the front of the ice chest/cabinet.

Mark all food varieties with the name and the date before freezing so they can be handily recognized.

Peruse more food stockpiling tips here.

3. Incorporate a portion of your number one dinner

Make a go-to rundown of dinners that you appreciate

Present new recipes when you have additional time

Ponder having a themed night, such as Meatless Monday for instance.

4. Go through your extras

Plan feasts that can be refrigerated and warmed up or eaten cold the following day, for example, pasta prepare, soup, shepherd's pie, curry, lasagna, or hamburger stew.

Utilize extra vegetables in an omelet, soup, or salad, or add extra meat to a curry or sautéed food.

Recall extras put away in the ice chest should be utilized in three days or less.

5. Cook in mass

Cook extra and refrigerate or freeze the extras. Pies, curries, stews, and goulashes all freeze well.

If you are utilizing the stove, ponder what else you can cook simultaneously. If you are doing a meal, you could cook a few chicken bosoms to go in sandwiches.

6. Make your fixings work

Pick recipes that utilization similar key fixings, for example, broiled chicken, chicken pan-fried food, and chicken sandwiches

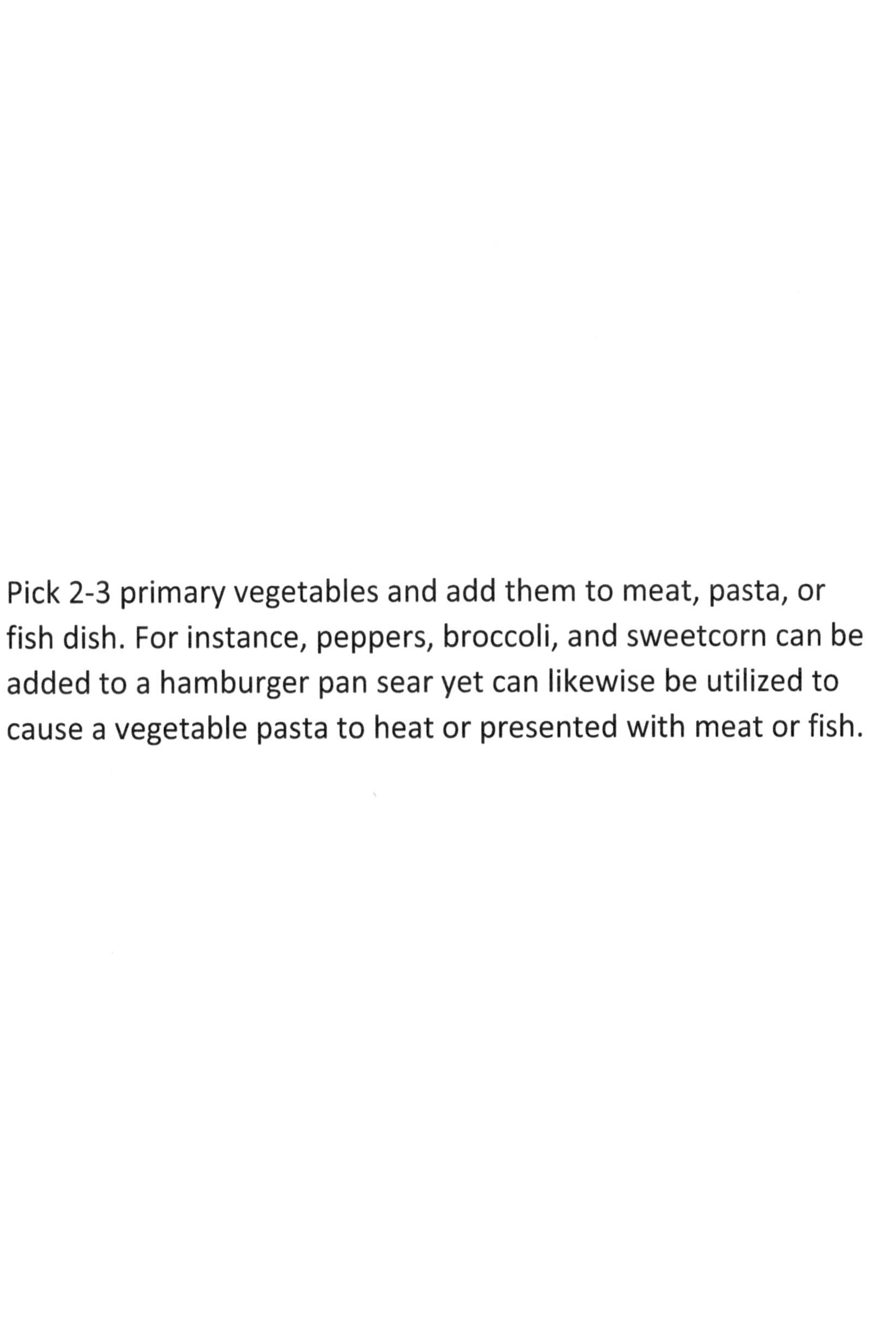

Pick 2-3 primary vegetables and add them to meat, pasta, or fish dish. For instance, peppers, broccoli, and sweetcorn can be added to a hamburger pan sear yet can likewise be utilized to cause a vegetable pasta to heat or presented with meat or fish.

CHAPTER SIX (6)

GUIDELINES TO KEEP OFF THE WEIGHT UNTIL THE END OF TIME

There's a superior method for getting thinner. These eating-less junk food tips can assist you with staying away from diet traps and making enduring weight reduction progress.

The young lady grinned while at the same time changing the shaft weight scale

What's the best eating routine for solid weight reduction?

Get any eating routine book and it will profess to hold every one of the responses to effectively losing all the weight you need — and keeping it off. In some cases, the key is to eat less and practice more, others that low fat is the best way to go, while others recommend removing carbs. Anyway, what would it be advisable for you to accept?

In all actuality there is no "one size fits all" answer for extremely durable solid weight reduction. What works for one individual may not work for you, since our bodies answer diversely to various food sources, contingent upon hereditary qualities and other wellbeing factors. Finding the strategy for weight reduction that is ideal for you will probably take time and require persistence, responsibility, and a few trials and error with various food sources and diets.

While certain individuals answer well to counting calories or comparable prohibitive techniques, others answer better to having more opportunities in arranging their get-healthy plans. Being free to just keep away from broiled food varieties or cut back on refined carbs can place them in a good position. Thus, don't get excessively deterred on the off chance that an eating routine that worked for another person doesn't work for you. What's more, don't thump yourself if an eating regimen demonstrates excessively prohibitive for you to stay with. At last, an eating routine is possibly ideal for you if it's one you can stay with over the long haul.

Keep in mind: while there's no simple fix to getting in shape, there are a lot of advances you can take to foster a better relationship with food, control profound triggers to gorging, and accomplish a sound weight.

Four famous weight reduction methodologies

1. Cut Calories

A few specialists accept that effectively dealing with your weight boils down to a basic condition: If you eat fewer calories than you consume, you get in shape. Sounds simple, correct? Why is getting in shape so hard?

Weight reduction is certainly not a direct occasion over the long haul. At the point when you cut calories, you might drop weight for the initial not many weeks, for instance, and afterward, something changes. You eat a similar number of calories yet you lose less weight or no weight by any means. That is because when you get in shape, you're losing water and lean tissue as well as fat, your digestion eases back, and your body changes in alternate ways. In this way, to keep dropping weight every week, you want to keep cutting calories.

A calorie isn't generally a calorie. Eating 100 calories of high fructose corn syrup, for instance, can distinctively affect your body more than eating 100 calories of broccoli. The stunt for supported weight reduction is to jettison the food sources that are loaded with calories however don't encourage you (like treats) and supplant them with food sources that top you off without being stacked with calories (like vegetables).

A significant number of us don't necessarily eat basically to fulfill hunger. We likewise go to nourishment for solace or to assuage pressure — which can rapidly crash any weight reduction plan.

2. Cut carbs

An alternate approach to reviewing weight reduction distinguishes the issue as not one of consuming such a large number of calories, yet rather how the body collects fat in the wake of consuming sugars — specifically the job of the chemical insulin. At the point when you eat a feast, sugars from the food enter your circulatory system as glucose. To hold your glucose levels in line, your body generally consumes this glucose before it consumes fat from a dinner.

If you eat a starch-rich dinner (bunches of pasta, rice, bread, or French fries, for instance), your body discharges insulin to assist with the flood of this glucose into your blood. As well as controlling glucose levels, insulin completes two things: It keeps your fat cells from delivering fat for the body to consume as fuel (because its need is to consume the glucose) and it makes more fat cells for putting away all that your body can't consume off. The outcome is that you put on weight and your body currently requires more fuel to consume, so you eat more. Since insulin just consumes sugars, you long for carbs thus starting an endless loop of consuming carbs and putting on weight. To get more fit, the thinking goes, you want to break this cycle by lessening carbs.

Carb cycle

Most low-carb eats less backer supplanting carbs with protein and fat, which could have some bad long-haul consequences for your wellbeing. If you truly do attempt a low-carb diet, you can lessen your dangers and cut off your admission of immersed and trans fats by picking lean meats, fish and vegan wellsprings of protein, low-fat dairy items, and eating a lot of verdant green and non-dull vegetables.

3. Cut fat

It's a pillar of many weights control plans: if you would rather not get fat, don't eat fat. Stroll down any supermarket walkway and you'll be barraged with diminished fat bites, dairy, and bundled feasts. In any case, while our low-fat choices have detonated, so have stoutness rates. All in all, why haven't low-fat eating regimens worked for a greater amount of us?

Not all fat is awful. Solid or "great" fats can assist with controlling your weight, as well as deal with your temperaments and battle weakness. Unsaturated fats found in avocados, nuts, seeds, soy milk, tofu, and greasy fish can assist with topping you off while adding a little delectable olive oil to a plate of vegetables, for instance, can make it more straightforward to eat good food and work on the general nature of your eating regimen.

We frequently make unacceptable compromises. A significant number of us wrongly trade fat for the unfilled calories of sugar and refined carbs. Rather than eating entire fat yogurt, for instance, we eat low-or no-fat adaptations that are loaded with sugar to compensate for the deficiency of taste. Or on the other hand, we trade our greasy breakfast bacon for a biscuit or doughnut that causes quick spikes in glucose.

4. Follow the Mediterranean eating routine

The Mediterranean eating routine underscores eating great fats and great carbs alongside enormous amounts of new products of the soil, nuts, fish, and olive oil — and just unassuming measures of meat and cheddar. However, the Mediterranean eating routine is something beyond food. Ordinary active work and imparting dinners to others are additionally significant parts.

Anything that weight reduction methodology you attempt, it's critical to remain propelled and keep away from normal counting calories entanglements, like close-to-home eating.

Control close-to-home eating

We don't necessarily eat essentially to fulfill hunger. Over and over again, we go to food when we're focused on or restless, which can wreck any eating routine and pack on the pounds. Do you eat when you're concerned, exhausted, or forlorn? Do you nibble before the TV toward the finish of an unpleasant day? Perceiving you're close to home eating triggers can have a significant effect on your weight reduction endeavors. Assuming that you eat when you're:

Focused - track down better ways of quieting yourself. Attempt yoga, reflection, or absorbing a hot shower.

Falling short on energy - find other mid-evening shots in the arm. Have a go at strolling around the block, paying attention to empowering music, or laying down for a brief rest.

Desolate or exhausted - contact others as opposed to going after the cooler. Call a companion who makes you chuckle, take your canine for a walk, or go to the library, shopping center, or park — anyplace there's kin.

Practice careful eating all things being equal

Keep away from interruptions while eating. Make an effort not to eat while working, sitting in front of the TV, or driving. It's excessively simple to gorge thoughtlessly.

Focus. Eat gradually, enjoying the scents and surfaces of your food. Assuming that your psyche meanders, tenderly return your regard for your food and how it tastes.

Shake things up to zero in on the experience of eating. Have a go at utilizing chopsticks instead of a fork, or utilize your utensils with your non-prevailing hand.

Quit eating before you are full. It requires investment for the sign to arrive at your cerebrum that you've had enough. Try not to feel committed to continue cleaning your plate.

Remain inspired

Long-lasting weight reduction requires rolling out solid improvements to your way of life and food decisions. To remain persuaded:

Track down a cheering segment. Social help implies a ton. Programs like Jenny Craig and Weight Watchers use bunch backing to affect weight reduction and deep-rooted good dieting. Search our help — whether as family, companions, or a care group — to get the consolation you want.

Steady-minded individuals will win in the end. Getting more fit too quickly can negatively affect your psyche and body, causing you to feel lazy, depleted, and wiped out. Expect to lose one to two pounds per week so you're losing fat as opposed to water and muscle.

Put forth objectives to keep you spurred. Momentary objectives, such as needing to squeeze into a swimsuit for the mid-year, generally don't function as well as needing to feel surer or become better for the good of your kids. At the point when allurement strikes, center around the advantages you'll harvest from being better.

Use devises to keep tabs on your development. Cell phone applications, wellness trackers, or just keeping a diary can assist you with monitoring the food you eat, the calories you consume, and the weight you lose. Seeing the outcomes in high contrast can assist you with remaining spurred.

Get a lot of rest. The absence of rest invigorates your hunger so you need more food than typical; simultaneously, it stops you from feeling fulfilled, making you need to continue to eat. Lack of sleep can likewise influence your inspiration, so go for the gold of value rest an evening.

Eliminate sugar and refined carbs

Whether you're explicitly meaning to cut carbs, the vast majority of us eat unfortunate measures of sugar and refined starches like white bread, pizza batter, pasta, cakes, white flour, white rice, and improved breakfast oats. However, supplanting refined carbs with their entire grain partners and wiping out sweets and treats is just essential for the arrangement. Sugar is concealed in food varieties as different as canned soups and vegetables, pasta sauce, margarine, and many decreased fat food sources. Since your body gets all, it needs from sugar normally happening in food, this additional sugar ends up being meaningless however a lot of void calories and undesirable spikes in your blood glucose.

Less sugar can mean a slimmer waistline

Calories got from fructose (found in sweet refreshments, for example, pop and handled food sources like doughnuts, biscuits, and candy) are bound to add to fat around your tummy. Scaling back sweet food varieties can mean a slimmer waistline as well as a lower hazard of diabetes.

Top off with the natural product, veggies, and fiber

Regardless of whether you're cutting calories, that doesn't guarantee to mean you need to eat less food. High-fiber food sources like the organic product, vegetables, beans, and entire grains are higher in volume and take more time to process, making them filling — and extraordinary for weight reduction.

It's by and large alright to eat as many new leafy foods and boring vegetables as you need — you'll feel full before you've gotten out of hand on the calories.

Eat vegetables crude or steamed, not broiled or breaded, and dress them with spices and flavors or a little olive oil for some zing.

Add natural products to low-sugar oat — blueberries, strawberries, and cut bananas. You'll in any case appreciate loads of pleasantness, yet with fewer calories, not so much sugar, but rather more fiber.

Mass out sandwiches by adding solid veggie decisions like lettuce, tomatoes, fledglings, cucumbers, and avocado.

Nibble on carrots or celery with hummus rather than fatty chips and plunge.

Add more veggies to your #1 primary course to make your dish more significant. Indeed, even pasta and sautés can be diet-accommodating assuming that you utilize not so many noodles but rather more vegetables.

Begin your feast with salad or vegetable soup to assist with topping you off so you eat less of your entrée.

Assume responsibility for your food climate

Put yourself in a position for weight reduction accomplishment by assuming responsibility for your food climate: when you eat, the amount you eat, and what food sources you make effectively accessible.

Cook your feasts at home. This permits you to control both piece size and what goes into the food. Eatery and bundled food sources for the most part contain much more sugar, unfortunate fat, and calories than food prepared at home — in addition, the piece sizes will quite often be bigger.

Serve yourself more modest parts. Utilize little plates, bowls, and cups to cause your segments to seem bigger. Try not to eat out of enormous dishes or straightforwardly from food holders, which makes it challenging to evaluate the amount you've eaten.

Eat early. Studies recommend that consuming a greater amount of your every day calories at breakfast and less at supper can assist you with dropping more pounds. Eating a bigger, sound breakfast can kick off your digestion, stop you from feeling hungry during the day, and give you additional opportunities to consume the calories.

Quick for 14 hours every day. Attempt to have supper before the day and afterward quick until breakfast the following morning. Eating just when you're most dynamic and offering your processing an extended reprieve might help weight reduction.

Plan your dinners and snacks somewhat early. You can make your little part snacks in plastic sacks or holders. Eating on a timetable will assist you with abstaining from eating when you're not eager.

Hydrate. Thirst can frequently be mistaken for hunger, so by drinking water, you can keep away from additional calories.

Limit how many enticing food varieties you have at home. If you share a kitchen with non-calorie counters, store liberal food sources hidden.

Get rolling

How much activity helps weight reduction is available to discuss, yet the advantages go far past copying calories. Exercise can expand your digestion and work on your viewpoint — and it's something you can profit from in the present moment. Take a walk, stretch, and move around and you'll have more energy and inspiration to handle different strides in your health improvement plan.

Need time for a long exercise? Three 10-minute sprays of activity each day can be similarly on a par with one 30-minute exercise.

Keep in mind: anything is better than a kick in the pants than nothing. Get going gradually with limited quantities of actual work every day. Then, at that point, as you begin to get in shape and have more energy, you'll find it simpler to turn out to be all the more truly dynamic.

Find the practice you appreciate. Take a stab at strolling with a companion, moving, climbing, cycling, playing Frisbee with a canine, partaking in a pickup round of ball, or playing action-based computer games with your children.

Keeping the load off

You might have heard the broadly cited measurement that 95% of individuals who shed pounds on a careful nutritional plan will recapture it inside a couple of years — or even months. While there isn't a lot of hard proof to help that case, the facts confirm that many weights reduction plans flop in the long haul. Frequently that is basically because abstaining from food that is too prohibitive is extremely difficult to keep up with over the long run. Notwithstanding, that doesn't mean your weight reduction endeavors are ill-fated to disappointment. A long way from it.

Since it was laid out in 1994, The National Weight Control Registry (NWCR) in the United States, has followed north of 10,000 people who have lost critical measures of weight and kept it off for significant periods. The investigation has discovered that members who've been fruitful in keeping up with their weight reduction share a few normal procedures. Anything that diet you use to get thinner in any case, embracing these propensities might assist you with keeping it off:

Remain truly dynamic. Fruitful health food nuts in the NWCR concentrate on practice for around an hour, ordinarily strolling.

Keep a food log. Recording what you eat consistently assists with keeping you responsible and propelled.

Have breakfast consistently. Most regularly in the review, it's an oat and organic product. Having breakfast helps digestion and fights off hunger later in the day.

Eat more fiber and less unfortunate fat than the ordinary American eating routine.

Consistently look at the scale. Gauging yourself week by week might assist you with distinguishing any little puts on in weight, empowering you to immediately make a restorative move before the issue raises.

Observe less TV. Scaling back the time spent sitting before a screen can be a vital piece of embracing a more dynamic way of life and forestalling weight gain.

www.ingramcontent.com/pod-product-compliance
Lightning Source LLC
LaVergne TN
LVHW052057160826
845678LV00015B/3271

* 9 7 9 8 8 4 6 3 6 9 6 1 0 *